Ready-To-Eat Healthy Convenience Foods

At Your U.S. Grocery Store

Author

amazon.com/author/paulachenderson

ISBN: 9798336165920

Front Cover designed by Paula C. Henderson
Lemon graphic by Tamalee on Pixabay
pixabay.com/illustrations/lemon-background-lemon-wallpaper-6712130/

Contents

1 CHAPTER ONE

Too busy to cook from scratch? But, you want to eat healthy? This is your go-to list of healthy, ready-to-eat foods you can find at your local grocery store and I've included some recipes too. This is for those days, those weeks, when you just can't think of anything for your next weeks menu.

Ready to Eat Healthy Foods From Your Grocery Store

I made you this list for those days when you just cannot think of anything to prepare and don't have much time but you want something healthy and quick. Who has time to cook from scratch?

When you are trying to put your grocery list together or a menu together and your mind goes blank. While I have fresh produce included because that is where you will find the healthiest foods, I wanted to include frozen and shelf-stable foods that you can keep on hand. Many of these foods will be familiar, but I hope, also, that you discover some new foods to look for in your local grocer.

Food companies have finally gotten the hint that many of us are looking for some quick **healthy** meals. You won't find any white potatoes or wheat pasta here as we are trying to limit those unhealthy high carbs. That doesn't mean there aren't some **healthy high-carb** foods so if you are watching your weight be mindful that otherwise healthy foods like sweet potatoes and legumes are high carbs. Also, note there are a few food items with cheese (dairy) but since they are covering vegetables we may have included a few for those of you who are trying to move toward a healthier diet or trying to get your kids to eat more vegetables but simply don't have time for a home-cooked meal from scratch.

For those avoiding gluten, dairy, nightshades, and soy here are some tips.

If you are avoiding nightshades you will want to avoid any food that has eggplant, tomatoes, white potatoes, hot peppers, bell peppers, tomatillos, and by-products of any of these foods like hot sauce or pimento.

Gluten is a grain and so, if you are avoiding grains you will also be avoiding gluten. Grains are corn, oats, wheat, and rice. All grains are high-carb foods. There are still misconceptions about gluten. I was at a friend's house and she said to me, "I have whole wheat bread for you since I know you are gluten-free." She was under the assumption gluten is strictly white bread and white flour. This is wrong. White and wheat flour are glutinous.

For those avoiding soy, I want to remind you that edamame beans are soybeans. Tofu is also soybeans.

BEVERAGES

Okay, maybe you are thinking that all beverages are quick, ready to use or consume. But, not all beverages are healthy.

Water. Water, of course, is your best beverage of choice and it is the one beverage you should drink more of than any other. I suggest getting into the habit of having water with your meals. Most medications, supplements, and over-the-counter meds are absorbed by the body much easier when taken with water unless otherwise instructed by your physician. If you find that water bothers your stomach, even the bottled water, even after trying various filters, I suggest trying Distilled Water. I buy it in gallon jugs and fill up my reusable water bottle, but Smart Water does offer single-serve plastic water bottles.

Juice. The first thing to remember about juice is that you should keep it to a minimum. Juice, although a natural sugar, is still a sugar and your body will react to it as it does any sugar. If and when you do choose a juice choose the "not-from-concentrate". Be sure it is actual juice and not a flavored drink. Always take note of the sugars and carbs on the label of any juice product or any smoothie that includes juice. It is because of this that I am not including juice or smoothies.

Did you know the average-size fresh orange has just 11 carbs, but a small 8-ounce glass of orange juice has around 26 carbs? Most people drink a 16-ounce glass of orange juice which has a whopping 47 carbs.

- Campbell's Tomato Juice (Nightshade Alert)
- Coconut Milk
- Coffee in limited amounts
- Lakewood Pure Celery Juice (Not From Concentrate)
- Unsweetened Almond Milk
- Unsweetened Tea (especially herbal tea)
- V-8 Original (Avoid this if you are avoiding nightshades)
- V-8 Low Sodium
- Water

FRESH FRUIT

Ready to eat fruit is of course very healthy. Great for breakfast or a snack. Most produce departments have pre-washed and pre-cut fruits and vegetables so look for those.

- Apples
- Banana
- Blackberries
- Blueberries
- Cantaloupe (find the one already cut up for you)
- Grapes
- Nectarines
- Orange
- Peaches
- Pears
- Pineapple Chunks that are ready to eat.
- Plum
- Raspberries
- Strawberries
- Watermelon (find the one already cut up for you)

FRESH Vegetables

A few of these may need to be peeled or sliced but many grocers now have vegetables already peeled and cut up for you to choose from. Look for those.

- Baby cut carrots
- Broccoli florets
- Broccoli Slaw
- Carrot sticks
- Cauliflower: great for any dip, hummus, or guacamole you like.
- Celery Sticks: I love the 4 packs of pre-cut celery sticks. There are three to four sticks in each sealed pack. So the other three packages stay fresh longer until you get ready to eat them.
- Chopped Salad Kit: Caesar Salad in a bag
- Classic Iceberg Salad
- Cucumbers
- Fajita mix: usually consist of pre-sliced peppers and onions
- Lettuce: all varieties
- Marketside Asian Chopped Salad Kit (bag)
- Marketside Butternut squash (bag, cubed)
- Marketside Chef Salad with Uncured Ham and Turkey
- Marketside Cobb Salad with Turkey and Uncured Bacon Salad
- Marketside Kale Pecan Cranberry Chopped Salad Kit (bag)
- Marketside Sunflower Bacon Crunch Chopped Salad Kit 10oz bag
- Mushrooms: all varieties
- Pre-made Salads in a bag. There are so many choices now. Romaine, Caesar, Kale Salad, Spinach, and many others come with dressings.
- Prepared salads
- Shredded Carrots
- Shredded Iceberg Lettuce
- Sliced Green Onions
- Snow Peas: like the sugar snap peas these are good with a dip, added to a salad or a stir-fry.
- Spinach in a bag: it's been washed!
- Squash – pre-sliced
- Sugar Snap Peas in a bag that has already been washed. These are a great snack with dip or added to a salad or stir-fry.

- Sweet Potatoes can be microwaved in a jiffy.
- Sweet Potato Cubes (in a bag)
- Taylor Farms BLT Salad with Chicken and Bacon
- Taylor Farms Caesar Salad with Bacon and Chicken
- Taylor Farms Ginger Garlic Stir Fry Kit (bag)
- Taylor Farms Roasted Red Pepper Hummus Snack Tray
- Taylor Farms Stir Fry Kit (bag) Brussels sprouts, broccoli stalk & florets, red cabbage, kale, carrot and pea pods
- Tomatoes
- Tri-color coleslaw – just add dressing
- Vegetable Medley: Broccoli florets, cauliflower florets, baby carrots. (bag)Great for soups, dips, stir-fry, or salads.
- Zucchini – pre-sliced

FROZEN VEGETABLES AND DINNERS

These vegetables have been washed and sliced and are ready to add to a dish or a microwave as a ready-made quick meal.

I wanted to separate these veggie pasta's from the rest of the list because they are very high carb. But, they are gluten-free and therefore healthier for those who are eating gluten-free. Most of these are made with legumes and some are pasta made using a combination of zucchini and legumes. They are very good, I've tried them! And quick and easy straight in and out of the microwave. I combine mine with ground beef, mixed vegetables, or frozen spinach and this lowers the per-serving carb amount.

- Birds Eye Veggie Pasta Penne with Cheddar Cheese Sauce (bag)
- Birds Eye Veggie Pasta Rotini Marinara
- Birds Eye Veggie Pasta, Rotini Alfredo

And now the main list of frozen vegetables and dinners

- Birds Eye Broccoli Tots
- Birds Eye Creamy Spinach Bake
- Birds Eye Crispy Cauliflower Florets
- Birds Eye Fire-Roasted Brussels Sprouts
- Birds Eye Fire Roasted Carrots
- Birds Eye Garlic Baby Peas and Mushrooms
- Birds Eye Maple Glazed Carrots
- Birds Eye Mashed Cauliflower Sour Cream and Chive
- Birds Eye Normandy Blend: Sliced Carrots, zucchini, yellow squash, broccoli and cauliflower florets
- Birds Eye Oven Roasters Broccoli & Cauliflower
- Birds Eye Oven Roasters Brussels Sprouts & Carrots
- Birds Eye Ranch Broccoli Florets
- Birds Eye Riced Cauliflower Spanish Style
- Birds Eye Seasoned Asian Medley
- Birds Eye Seasoned Brown Sugar Sweet Potatoes

- Birds Eye Seasoned Garlic Cauliflower
- Birds Eye Skillets Balsamic Brussels Sprouts
- Birds Eye Skillets Garlic & Wine Mushrooms
- Birds Eye Skillets Garlic Butter Green Beans
- Birds Eye Skillets Sesame Broccoli
- Birds Eye Steamfresh Asparagus Spears
- Birds Eye Steamfresh Carrots, Broccoli and Cauliflower
- Birds Eye Steamfresh Mixed Vegetables
- Birds Eye Steamfresh Whole Green Beans
- Birds Eye Steamfresh: broccoli, carrots, sugar snap peas & water chestnuts
- Caulipower Real Cluckin Chicken (chicken tenders breaded with low-carb cauliflower)
- Cut Okra (ready to drop in your next minestrone or gumbo)
- Diced Avocados (frozen)
- Frozen Broccoli Stir Fry
- Great Value Seasoning Blend with diced onions, celery, red peppers, green peppers, and parsley flakes. (bag)
- Green Giant Restaurant Style Asparagus Roasted Red Potatoes & Onions: one of the very few items included with potatoes since it has asparagus and onions and no cheese sauce.
- Green Giant Restaurant Style Garlic Parmesan Green Beans
- Green Giant Riced Veggies Cauliflower Medley: eat as is or add ground beef or even breakfast sausage crumbles.
- Green Giant Simply Steam Broccoli & Cheese Sauce 10-ounce bag
- Green Giant Simply Steam Broccoli, Carrots, Cauliflower & Cheese Sauce
- Green Giant Simply Steam Garlic & Herb Vegetable Medley
- Green Giant Simply Steam Mediterranean Blend
- Green Giant Simply Steam Tuscan Seasoned Broccoli
- Green Giant Veggie Fries Zucchini Garlic & Parmesan
- Green Giant Veggie Spirals Zucchini
- Green Giant Veggie Tots Broccoli & Cheese
- Marketside Asian Chopped Salad Kit
- Riced Cauliflower: just mix straight from the freezer for a cold salad like frozen peas, riced cauliflower and toss with dressing. Or, use your microwave to heat quickly. Of course, this can also

be used in oven casseroles and the skillet for quick stir frys or soups.

- Tasty Bite Protein Bowls (these are VERY high in carbs but the ingredients list reads very healthy. For example, the Mediterranean-style variety ingredients list includes Water, chickpeas, couscous, vinaigrette, carrots, red bell pepper, red kidney beans, navy beans, and black beans.) As you can imagine from the ingredients list this is also very high in fiber!

FROZEN FRUIT

Frozen fruit is plentiful and will, of course, last longer than fresh fruit. It does change the texture but if you are okay with that then try them all. I like to set a serving size out in the refrigerator the night before if I am planning on having some for breakfast. But, if I take my lunch I know it will thaw come lunch time in my lunch bag but still be cold.

- Berry Medley
- Cherry Berry Blend
- Dark Sweet Cherries, Pitted
- Mango Chunks
- Mixed fruit
- Pineapple Chunks
- Sliced Bananas
- Sliced Peaches
- Sliced Strawberry Banana Blend (bag)
- Whole Strawberries

JARS AND CANS

- Artichokes
- Aunt Nellie's Red Cabbage (jar)
- Avocado Oil
- Bamboo Shoots
- Beets
- Broth
- Bruschetta
- Cocktail onions
- Coconut Oil
- Green Beans
- Hearts of Palm
- Italian Mix Giardiniera
- Kimchi
- Legumes
- Margaret Holmes Squash with Vidalia Onions (can)
- Marinated Mushrooms
- Minced Garlic
- Olive Oil
- Olives: all varieties
- Pearl onions
- Peas
- Pesto
- Pickled asparagus
- Pickled green beans
- Pickled Okra
- Read 3 bean salad
- Refried Beans
- Roasted Red Pepper Strips
- Sauerkraut
- Spice World Easy Onion (looks like the jars of minced garlic)
- Spinach
- Sun-Dried Tomatoes
- Turnip greens
- Yams

MEATS AND SEAFOOD (Canned, Pouches and Jars)

- Anchovies
- Bumble Bee Applewood Smoke tuna (pouch)
- Bumble Bee Lemon Sesame & Ginger Tuna pouch
- Bumble Bee Mediterranean Herbs & Spices tuna(pouch)
- Canned chicken
- Canned roast beef
- Canned salmon
- Canned tuna
- Clams
- Great Value Pulled Pork in BBQ Sauce (Ingredients: pork, water, sugar, tomato paste, distilled vinegar, less than 2% of food starch salt, corn starch, Worcestershire sauce, and distilled vinegar.)
- John Soules Foods Chicken Fajitas (pouch)
- Keystone Canned Beef (Ingredients: Beef, Sea salt.)
- Keystone Canned Ground Beef (Ingredients: Beef, sea salt)
- Oysters
- Starkist Chunk Light Tuna in water (pouch)
- StarKist Tuna Creations Herb and Garlic tuna pouch
- Starkist Tuna Creations Ranch (pouch)
- StarKist Tuna Creations, Lemon Pepper (pouch)

PREPARED FOODS MISCELLANEOUS

- Guacamole
- Peeled Hard Boiled Eggs (ready to eat. You'll find them near the eggs and butter) (bagged)
- Hummus
- Prepared Salads
- Roasted Chicken
- Sushi
- Veggie trays

Shelf Stable Heat-and-Eat

Reese Indian Style Cauliflower Harvest Bowl (Ingredients: Cauliflower, red pepper, olive oil, garlic, curry paste, ginger, salt, potassium chloride salt, lactic acid, white wine vinegar, and natural flavors.)

Pacific Foods Organic Roasted Red Pepper and Tomato Soup (shelf stable carton) (Ingredients: reduced fat milk, water, tomato paste, red bell peppers, sugar, roasted red bell peppers, roasted garlic, salt, butter, sodium citrate, nonfat dry milk, rice flour, garlic powder, onion powder, spices.)

Pacific Foods Organic Butternut Squash Soup (shelf-stable carton) (Ingredients: Butternut Squash Puree, water, soy base [water and soybeans], sugar, canola oil, salt, rice flour, spices, natural flavoring, onion powder, garlic powder.)

HEALTHY SNACKS

Vegetables, fruit, and nuts are your best choice for a snack. But here are some other great choices you can keep on hand.

- Great Value Trail Mix Omega-3 (If you can find a similar combination of ingredients in another brand that would be fine too) This product has zero sodium and just 11 carbs per serving. (Ingredients: dried cranberries, walnuts, pepitas, almonds, pecans, vegetable oil)

- KIND Dark Chocolate Nuts & Sea Salt Snack Bar (granola bar) (Ingredients: Almonds, peanuts, chicory, root fiber, honey, palm kernel oil, sugar, glucose syrup, rice flour, unsweetened chocolate, alkalized cocoa, salt, soy lecithin, natural flavor, and cocoa butter. Each bar has 16 carbs and 7 grams of fiber with Sodium at 140 mg.

I love foods prepared with Almond flour as it is a good source of protein and very low carb.

- Simple Mills Almond Flour Crackers Fine Ground Sea Salt: (ingredients: Almond flour, sunflower seeds, flax seeds, tapioca starch, cassava, organic sunflower oil, salt, organic onion, organic garlic, rosemary extract.)

The Simple Mills brand has many varieties of snack crackers made with Almond flour and other natural ingredients.

MENU IDEAS

BREAKFAST

I will sometimes wrap a sweet potato in foil and place it in my crockpot on low before bed. It's ready when I get up in the morning. I just add some butter and cinnamon/sugar. This makes a nice hot breakfast. Of course, you could also use the microwave in the morning if you prefer.

Those boiled eggs in the dairy section of your grocery store that have already been cooked and peeled are also a great choice. And there isn't anything wrong with an egg salad sandwich for breakfast if that sounds good to you. Just mix with some mayo, salt, and pepper and you are good to go!

The healthiest thing you could choose for breakfast is Nuts and seeds, maybe a small amount of fruit, and a glass of Unsweetened Vanilla Almond Milk. One thing I enjoy is slicing a banana into a bowl, tossing in some trail mix (nuts and seeds), and pouring Almond Milk on top. Grab a spoon and eat it like cereal. This is a very satisfying breakfast and very healthy.

Here are some HEALTHY quick, 10-30 minute menu ideas and recipes.

Chicken And Salsa

- One jar of your favorite salsa
- Skinless Boneless Chicken

You can bake a couple of chicken breasts in just 20 minutes or you can buy the cooked rotisserie chicken at the grocer's deli. They now sell it already removed from the bone and ready to eat. That would work great in this dish.

Just put the cooked, chopped, or shredded chicken with the salsa in a large skillet over medium heat. Stir around on occasion and heat through. Should only take five to ten minutes. Serve over a bed of lettuce, rice, and black beans, or warm some tortillas and make a soft taco.

Frozen Mushrooms And Ground Beef

- Birds Eye skillets Garlic and Wine Frozen Mushrooms
- One pound of ground beef

Variations: Add Frozen peas, mixed vegetables, riced cauliflower, or frozen chopped spinach

Brown the ground beef in a skillet and add the frozen Birds Eye Skillets Garlic and Wine Mushrooms. Go ahead and add any other vegetable you might like. Heat through and serve!

Ground Beef and Green Bean Skillet

- One pound of ground beef
- One can of French-style green beans (drained)

Brown the ground beef in a skillet. Drain one can of French-style green beans and add to the cooked ground beef.
Salt and pepper to taste.

This is a simple but satisfying meal. Affordable, no carbs and protein. If you wanted you could add a chopped tomato or a can of tomatoes.

Shrimp And Riced Cauliflower

- One bag of Frozen Raw Peeled, Deveined, Tail-Off Shrimp
- One bag of frozen riced cauliflower
- Chicken Bouillon (half cup prepared)
- Garlic Powder
- Frozen Peas
- Lemon Juice
- One tablespoon butter

Pour half a cup chicken bouillon into a skillet. Heat to med-high. Add frozen riced cauliflower and ½ teaspoon garlic powder. Bring to a boil. Add butter, shrimp, and peas. Cook for about five minutes. Add a tablespoon of lemon juice. Cover with a lid, turn the heat down to low. Cook an additional five minutes.

Lettuce

Include salad (any variety) in any and every dish you can. For years people ignored the benefits of iceberg lettuce saying, "It's nothing but water".

News Flash! Water is healthy for you. Lettuce, like iceberg and others that contain a lot of water our very hydrating for the body. Plus, they have nutrients too. Yes, even iceberg.

There are many varieties of lettuce with different taste profiles and different textures. Choose which one works best for however you plan to use it.

Iceberg lettuce, crisp and wet goes well on tacos or on top of burritos, baked chicken, shredded chicken, hamburgers, and sandwiches.

Romaine, everyone's favorite, goes well as the base of any salad you are building. Also goes great **under** lots of favorite foods like baked chicken, black beans, red beans, taco meat (think taco salad), and Caesar salad! Have you ever tried the lettuce bun? I find the iceberg lettuce leaves work best. Layer maybe two large leaves and use them as a bun. Just try it at least once. Most people are surprised at how much they like it and realize they don't miss the bread at all.

I encourage you to try all the different types of lettuce. They do not all taste the same and neither do they have the same texture.

Vegetables

Adopting a new rule for your ratio of vegetables to any other food on your plate is one of the healthiest choices you can make.

Traditionally, when we have pasta with vegetables say it's pasta primavera we have way more pasta than vegetables. Even when we have a protein and a side dish, our protein, such as fish, chicken, beef, or pork, is traditionally a larger portion than the vegetable on our plate.

A healthier ratio would be to make sure you are eating a very small serving of meat or pasta, rice or beans and the largest portion of your food is a vegetable like green beans, asparagus, brussels sprouts, squash, zucchini, broccoli, cauliflower, greens, salad or any other of the many, many vegetables available.

Vegetables are so versatile! You can eat them raw, in salads, with dip, as a stir-fry (quick meal idea), roasted in the oven, sautéed, in soup, boiled, mashed, in an omelet, as a side dish, or as your main dish.

Healthy Tips

Start drinking water with your meals.

Eat less overly processed foods and instead lean toward fresh unprocessed foods as often as possible.

If you are trying to cut down on your sugar don't substitute other sweeteners. Instead, eat less foods that taste sweet.

Did you know eating overly processed foods can cause faux hunger pangs? This is why people who eat fresh, unprocessed foods can eat less without feeling hungry.

I encourage you to try new foods. One year I tried one new food each week. Or, an old food I had tried before but didn't like, prepared differently.

ABOUT THE AUTHOR

amazon.com/author/paulachenderson

9 798336 165920